MENTAL HEALTH EDUCATION

An Effort to Educate People about Mental Health and Mental Illness.

Part-1

DAIRY NUMBER: 10286/2019-CO/L

Dr. Amit Phillora

&

Aleya Khan (Co-Author)

Every day begins with an act of courage and hope: getting out of bed

—Mason cooley

This book is dedicated to my Parents and fellow medical friends.

Preface

The Need for This Book:

The purpose of the book was to educate people about mental health education. The book explains different what is mental health is and what is mental illness is. The book explains different types of mental health illness. The book explains common mental illness like:

1. Depression;
2. Suicide Risk Assessment;
3. Substance Abuse
4. Anxiety Management Disorder;
5. Stress and Post Traumatic Stress Disorder;
6. Eating Disorder;
7. Schizophrenia.
8. Dementia.
9. Alzheimer.

Focus:

The focus of this book is to educate people about Mental Health illness.

Organization of the Text:

The book is divided into 3 sections:

Section A: Will have following topics:
1. Introduction to Mental Health and illness;
2. Depression.

Section B: Will have following topics:

3. Substance Abuse;
4. Anxiety Disorder Management.

Section C: Will have the following topics:

5. Stress and Post Traumatic Stress Disorder;
6. Eating Disorder.

Section D: Will have following topic:

7. Schizophrenia.
8. Dementia.
9. Alzheimer.

Highlights of the Book:

The key highlights of this book can be outlined as follows:

1. Introduction to Mental Health Illness;
2. Symptoms;
3. Cases.

This book will also serve as a desk reference for students and interns of psychology who are studying Bachelors, Masters and Diploma in Psychology because it has an optimum blend of theory as well practical. We sincerely believe that the readers will find the information being presented very useful.

Acknowledgements:

This book delves into the extensive literature that has already developed by eminent academicians, practitioners and researchers. The author acknowledges them for their works and ideologies incorporated in this volume.

Dr. Amit Phillora expresses his heartfelt gratitude to Dr. Ratna Johri, Coordinator in Indira Gandhi Open University, Jabalpur, an expert in Counselling Psychology.

He is extremely thankful to Group Captain (Retd.) BS Phillora, Dean of Studies, Engineering Staff College of India (ESCI) for guidance and valuable support in writing this informative book.

He is extremely thankful to Miss Shalini, Psychologist in Department of Dementia, at Nizam Institute of Medical Science (Hyderabad).

I am indebted to Dr. Shilpa Sharma Pandey, Medical Officer, Community Health Center, Kollar, Bhopal (MP) and Dr. Supriya Sharma MD (Pharmacology), Assistant Professor in Netaji Subhash Chandra Bose Medical College, Bhopal for clarifying conceptual issues related to Mental Health Education and Illness.

I am extremely thankful to Miss Aleya Khan, Global Goodwill Ambassador - in Canada, who gave me an opportunity to work in her Health Care Campaign Program in India, in February and May 2019, which gave me excellent exposure on some important and practical issues related to mental health education.

The author acknowledges, along with the publishers, the following reviewers for their invaluable feedback without which this book would have not come out in its present shape:

1. Mrs. Bhavani Sr. Counsellor in Sudisha Counseling Central, Hyderabad.
2. Dr. Seema Sharma, Head of Department (Botany), RDPG, Mandla.
3. Dr. Rama Gupta, Associate Professor (Botany), RDPG, Mandla.
4. Dr. Vandana, Post-Doctoral Fellowship (UGC), Pt. S.N.S University, Shahdol.
5. Dr. Sangeeta Mashih, Professor, Pt. S.N.S University, Shahdol.
6. Dr. Ashish Sharma, Sr. Lecturer, University of Management, Jabalpur.
7. Saurabh Pandey (Research Scholar), Assistant Professor (Electronic & Communication): Laxmi Narayan Institute of Technology Bhopal.
8. Dr. Suresh Naidu, Business Economics, Osmania University.
9. Dr. Aparna Chakrabarti, Head of Department, Library, Osmania University.
10. Dr. PK Jhinge, Principal, Jabalpur Engineering College.
11. Dr. Sheshpal Namdeo, Assistant Professor, Management, APS University Rewa.
12. DD Sharma, Former Joint Director Social Welfare and Panchayat Raj. Government of Madhya Pradesh.
13. Mr. Anil Senior Coordinator, IGNOU, Hyderabad.
14. Dr. Ratnakar, Director and owner of IMRF.
15. Miss Prabhjot Kaur, Asst.Professor, Communication Development (Delhi University).

The author also acknowledges the team of Kindle Direct Publishing for helping me in publishing the book.

Mental Health

A brief Introduction to this book

It's a textbook designed to generate awareness among the people and educating people what mental health is and what is mental illness. The book is divided into 3 parts. Each part will explain 2 sets of illness for mental health disorders. The book will explain what mental illness is, its symptoms and if it has a cure then explanation of the cure.

The most widely known mental illness are:

1. Depression;
2. Suicide;
3. Anxiety disorder;
4. Schizophrenia disorder;
5. Substance abuse;
6. Eating disorders.
7. Dementia
8. Alzheimer

We will explain each kind, its symptoms and treatment in this book.

Mental Health © 2019 by Dr. Amit Phillora. All Rights Reserved.
10286/2019-CO/L

All rights reserved. No part of this book may be reproduced in any form or by any electronic or mechanical means including information storage and retrieval systems, without permission in writing from the author. The only exception is by a reviewer, who may quote short excerpts in a review.

Cover designed by Cover Creator tool of KDP

This book is a work of mental Health Education. Mental health Illness, Symptoms, Cure, and treatment.

Dr. Amit Phillora
Visit my website at amazon.com/author/dr.amitphillora
Miss Aleya Khan

Through Kindle Direct Publishing.

CONTENTS

Preface 4
Acknowledgements: 7
Mental Health 9
Chapter-1: Mental Health 13
Chapter 2: Introduction to Depression 20
Chapter-3: Suicide Risk Assessment 36

Chapter-1: Mental Health

This is the Book Epigraph. Introduce your book with a quote, phrase, excerpt, poem, or verse that sets the stage for your book. It should always start on a new page. Use the attribution to tell readers where the quote comes from or who originally said it.

—Juliette Lewis

Introduction to Mental health:

"The bravest thing I ever did was continuing my life when I wanted to die." — Juliette Lewis.

Let us understand that what is mental health meaning is.

Mental health is often used as a substitute for mental health conditions- like:
- Depression;
- Anxiety conditions;
- Schizophrenia
- & Others.

According to World Health Organization(WHO), however, the mental health is a "state of well being in which every individual realizes his/her own potential, can cope with stresses of life, can work productively and fruitfully and is able to make a contribution to his or her community.

So, rather than being about what's the problem?" It is about "what's going well"

Stress can be measured by a psychometric instrument called "PERCEIVED STRESS SCALE" (PSS) which was designed by "Sheldon Cohen".

Based the results stress management plans can be designed by the psychologist for his/her patients.

Mental Health is about wellness rather than illness.

The benefit of being well:

To make things a bit clearer, some experts have tried coming up with different terms to explain the difference between "mental health" and "mental health conditions."

Phrases such as 'good mental health', 'positive mental health', 'mental wellbeing ', subjective wellbeing' and 'even happiness' and even wellness rather than illnesses. Some practitioners say that this is helpful whereas some disagree with this. They argue on the fact that using more words to describe mental health will create confusion.

Due to this others have tried to explain the difference by talking about a continuum where mental health is at one end of the spectrum - represented by feeling good & functioning well – while mental illness are the other-represented by symptoms that affects people's thoughts, feelings or thinking process.

Research shows that high levels of mental health are associated with:
1. Increased learning;
2. Increased creativity;
3. Increased productivity;
4. Good Pro-social behaviour;
5. Positive relationship with improved physical health and life expectancy.

In contrast mental health condition or mental illness can cause:
1. Distress;
2. Impact on day to day functioning and relationships
3. Poor physical health;
4. Pre-mature death from suicide.

It is important to know that mental health illness is complex and is a complicated situation. If a person is showing all symptoms of healthiness that doesn't mean that he is mentally healthy. There are chances of being diagnosed with mental illness with feeling well in many aspects of life.

Mental health is about:
1. Being cognitively healthy.
2. Being Emotionally healthy;
3. Being Socially healthy.

Symptoms for mental health conditions/illness:
Signs and symptoms of illness may vary, depending on the type of disorder, circumstance and other factors. Mental health conditions symptoms can affect:
1. Emotions;
2. Thoughts and Thinking Process;
3. Behaviours.

https://www.youtube.com/watch?v=6kaCdrvNGZw&feature=youtu.be

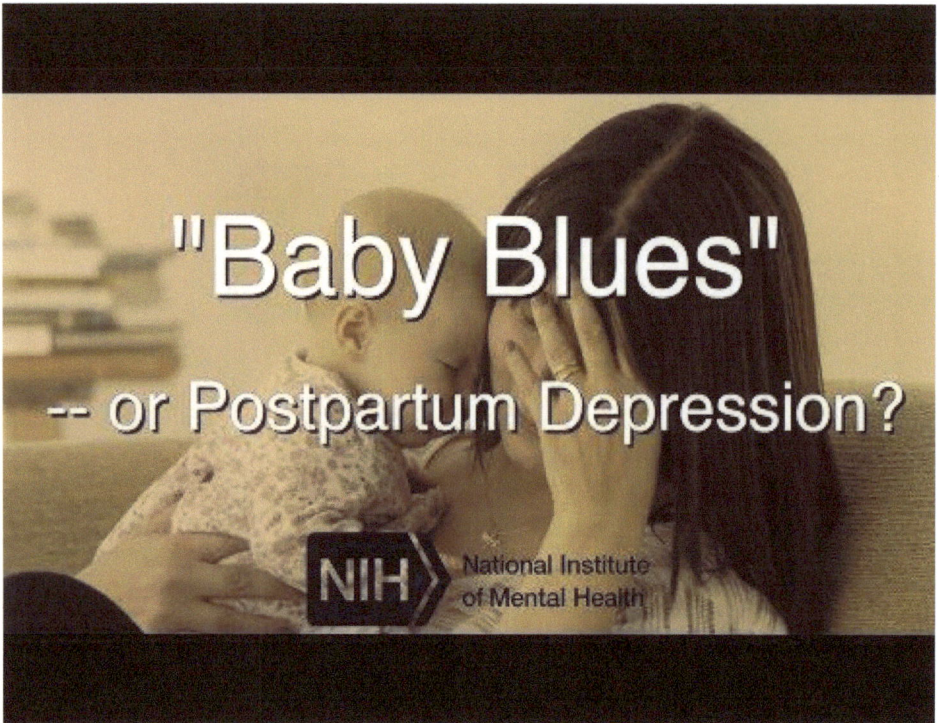

Examples of signs and symptoms include:

- Feeling Sad or Down
- Confused thinking or reduced ability to concentrate
- Excessive fears or worries, or extreme feeling of guilt;
- Mood Swings
- Making self-isolated;
- Low energy, laziness, problem in sleeping;
- Inability to cope up with stress or inability to perform daily tasks;
- Alcohol or drug abuse;
- Major changes in eating habits;
- Major changes in eating habits;
- Sex drive changes;
- Suicide thinking

Sometimes symptoms of mental health condition appear as physical problems such as stomach-ache, back ache, headache, or other unexplained pains or aches.

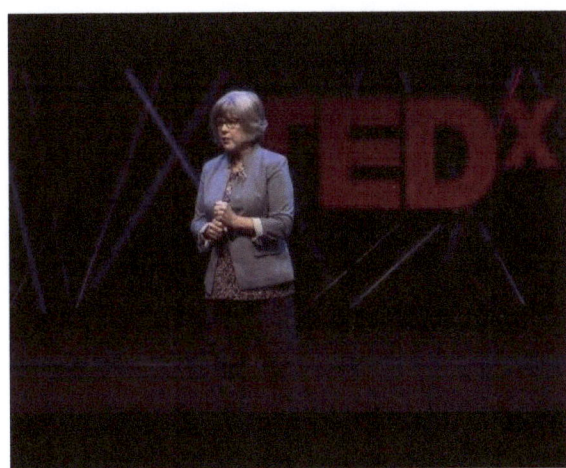

Mental Illness by kitty westin:
https://www.youtube.com/watch?v=OsRF8xGgbPA&feature=youtu.be

What Causes Mental Health illness?

Mental health illnesses, in general are thought to be caused by a variety of genetic and environmental factors:

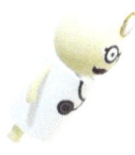

- **Inherited traits:** Mental illness is more common in people whose blood relatives also have a mental illness. That is it occurs due to genetic disorder in family as well. Certain genes may increase the risk of developing mental illness and your life situation may trigger it.
- **Environmental Exposures before birth:** Exposure to environmental stressors, inflammatory conditions, toxins, alcohol or drugs while in the womb can sometimes be linked with mental illness.
- **Brain Chemistry:** Neurotransmitters are naturally occurring brain chemicals that carry signals to other parts of your brain and body. When the neural networks involving these chemicals are impaired, the function of nerve system change, leading to depression.

△ △ △

Risk Factors:

Certain factors may increase the risk of developing mental illness. Few of the risk factors are mentioned below:
1. Having blood relative, such as parent or sibling, with mental illness;
2. Stressful life such as financial crisis, loss of loved one, death, divorce or separation;
3. An ongoing (chronic) medical conditions, such as diabetics, thyroid etc;
4. Post-Traumatic Stress Disorder (PTSD);
    a. Brain damage as a result of a serious injury (traumatic brain injury);
    b. Traumatic experience like military combat or being assaulted;
    c. Use of alcohol or recreational drugs;
    d. Being abused or neglected child;
    e. Middle child syndrome;
    f. Having few friends or few healthy relationships;
    g. A previous mental illness.

Complications related to Mental health:

Mental illness is a leading cause of disability. Unrelated mental illness can cause severe emotional, behavioural and physical health problems.

Complications sometimes linked to mental illness include:
1. Unhappiness and decreased enjoyment of the life;
2. Family condition;
3. Relationship difficulties;
4. Social isolation;
5. Problems with tobacco, alcohol and other drugs;
6. Missed work or school or other drugs;
7. Missed work, school or other problems related to work or school;
8. Legal and financial problem;
9. Poverty and homelessness;
10. Self-harm and harm to others, including homicide or suicide;
11. Week immune systems;
12. Heart disease and other medical illness.

Prevention

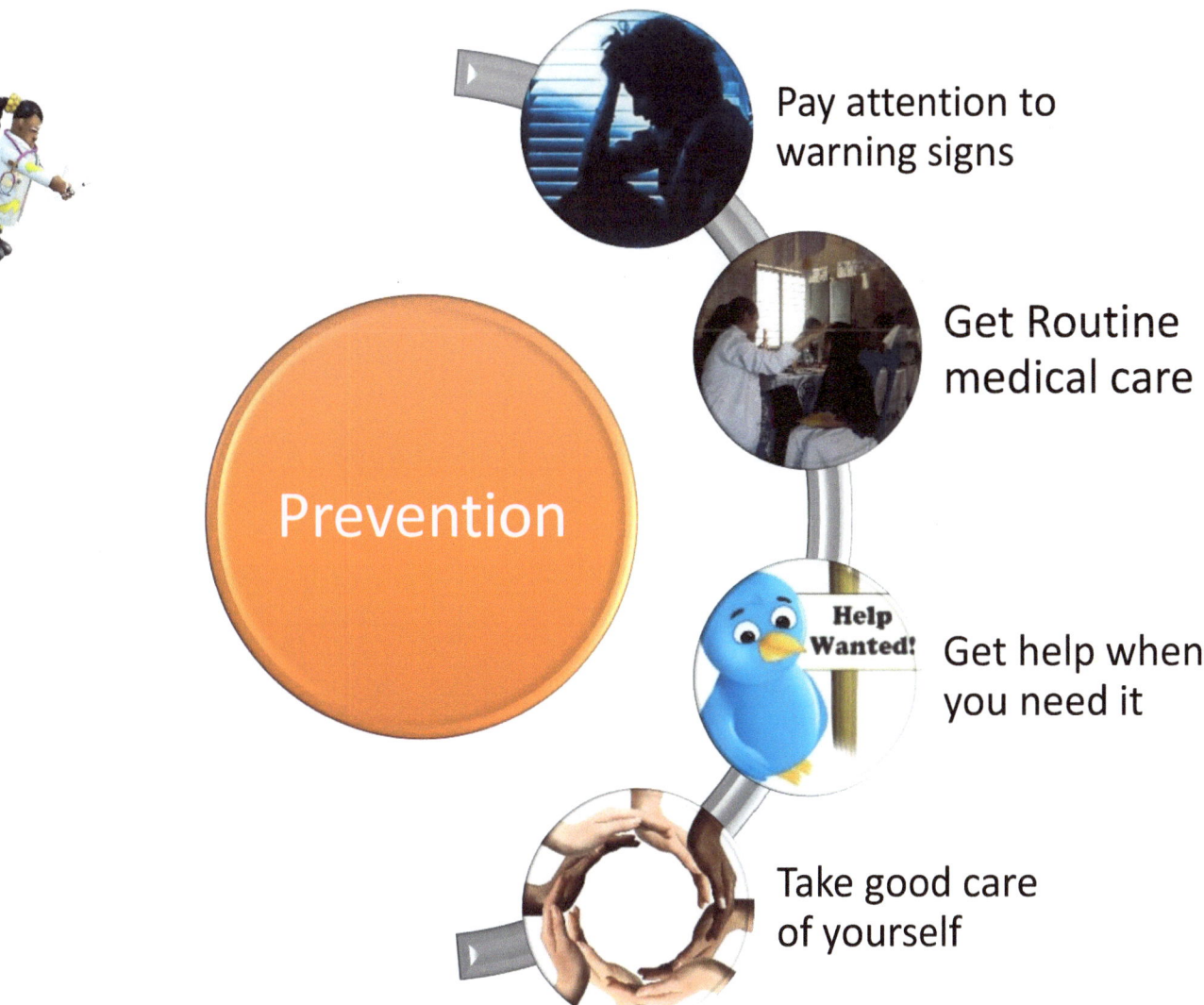

Chapter 2: Introduction to Depression

"There are wounds that never show on the body that are deeper and more hurtful than anything that bleeds."
—*Laurell K. Hamilton, Mistral's Kiss*

Depression (major depression) is common and serious medical illness that negatively affects how you feel, the way you think and how you act.

Fortunately, its treatable disorder. Depression caused feelings of sadness and or loss of interest in activities once enjoyed. It can lead to a variety of emotional and physical problems and can decrease a person's ability to function at work or at home.

Depression symptoms can vary from mild to severe and can include:
1. Feeling sad or having a depressed mood;
2. Loss of interest or pleasure in activities once enjoyed;
3. Changes in appetite – weight loss or gain unrelated to dieting;
4. Trouble sleeping or sleeping too much;
5. Loss of energy or increased fatigue;
6. Increase in purposeless physical activity;
7. Feeling worthless or guilty;
8. Difficulty in thinking, concentrating or making decision;
9. Thought of death or suicide.

Symptoms must last at least 2 weeks for diagnosis of depression.

Also, medical conditions (e.g. thyroid problems, a brain tumour or vitamin deficiency) can mimic symptoms of depression so it's important to rule out general medical causes.

Depression affects 1 in 15 adults (6.7%) in a given year. And 1 in 6 people (16.6%) will experience depression at some time in their life. Depression can strike at any time, but on average it first appears during late teens to mid-20s.

Women are most likely than men to experience depression. Some studies show that 1/3rd of women will experience a major depressive episode in their lifetime.

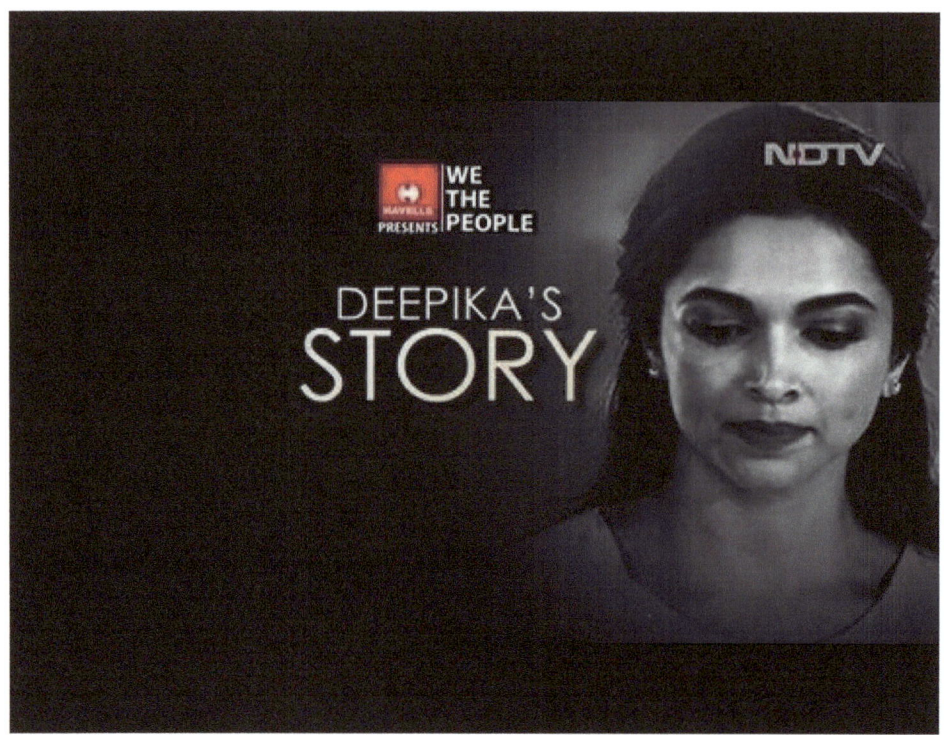

Deepika Padukone's Story | Interview | NDTV
https://www.youtube.com/watch?v=srGbyn8Ad5E&feature=youtu.be

Depression – Cause & Treatment:

Comorbidity refers to the presence of more than one diagnosis in an individual at the same time. Something that occurs together with high degree.

Depression and Anxiety go hand in hand and cannot be distinguished.

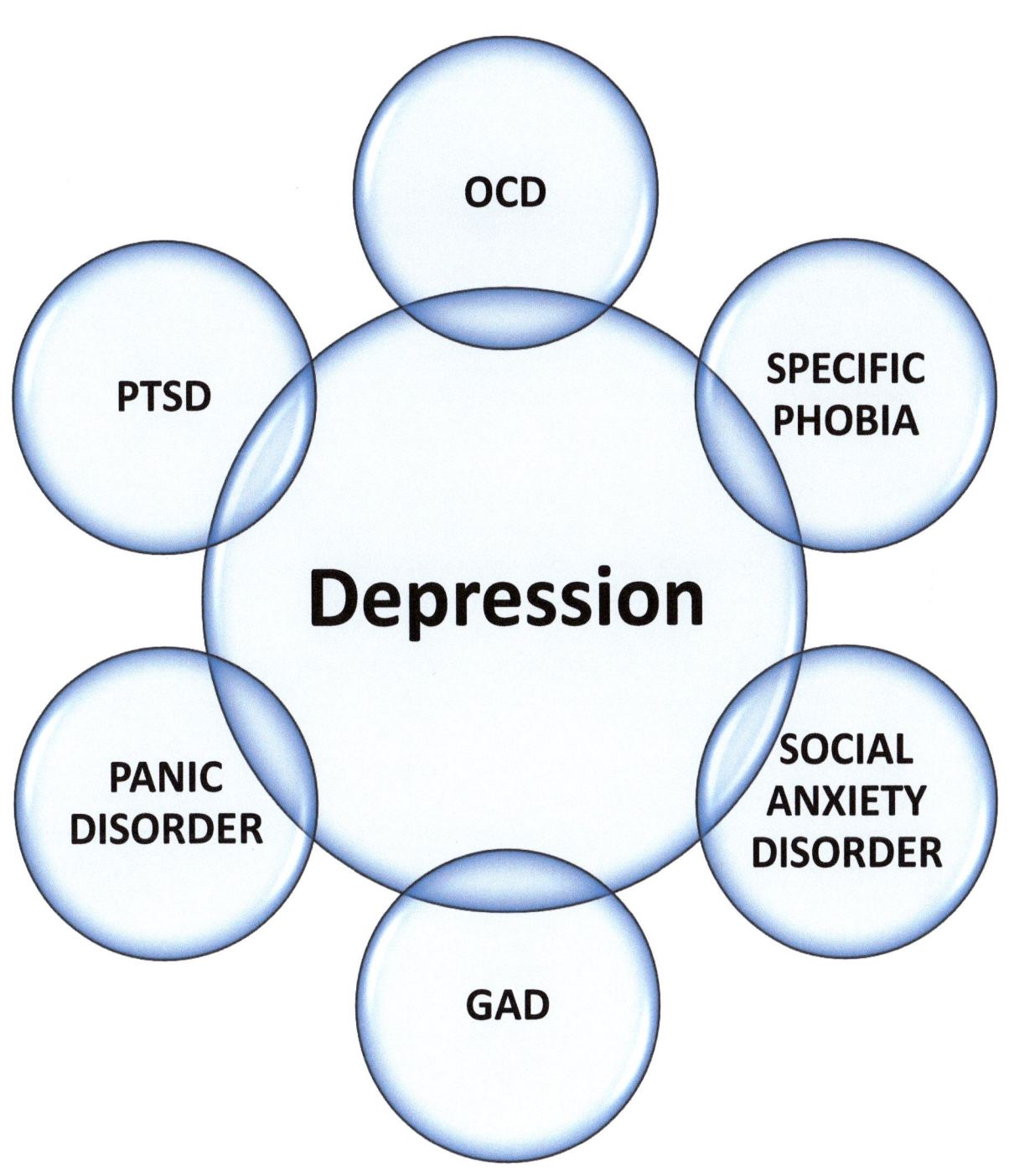

Depression is different from Sadness or Grief/Bereavement

The death of loved one, loss of a job or ending of a relationship are difficult experiences for a person to endure. It is normal for feelings of sadness or grief to develop in response to such situations. Those experiencing loss may often referred to as depressed.

But being sad is not the same as having depression. The grieving process is natural and unique to each individual and shares some of the same features of depression.

But being sad is not the same as having depression. The grieving process is natural and unique to each individual and shares some of the same features as that of depression.

However, there are few ways by which we can try to differentiate Sadness and Depression.
1. In grief, painful feelings come in waves, often intermixed with positive memories of deceased person. In major depression, mood &/or interest (pleasure) are decreased for most of the 2 weeks.
2. In grief, self-esteem is usually maintained. In major depression, feeling of worthlessness and self-loathing are common.
3. For some people, the death of a loved one can bring on major depression. Losing a job or being a victim of physical assault, or a major disaster can lead to depression for some people

When grief and depression co-exist or stays together then grief is more severe and last longer then grief without depression.

Despite some overlaps between grief and depression, they are both different. If you can distinguish between them then you will be able to help the person accurately and properly.

Depression – Risk factors:
1. **Biochemistry:** Differences in certain chemicals in the brain may cause depression;
2. **Genetics:** It can run in families;
3. **Personality:** People with low self-esteem, who are easily overwhelmed by stress or who are generally pessimistic appears to be more likely to get experienced with depression.
4. **Environmental Factors:** Continuous exposure to violence, neglect or abuse or poverty can also cause depression in some people.

Causes for Depression:
1. Genetic;
2. Neurotransmitters disturbances;
3. Psychosocial factors
    - Adverse experiences in childhood
    - Chronic major difficulties
    - Undesirable life events
    - Limited social networks

- Low self esteem

Few Of The Examples Of Physical Illness Due To Depression:

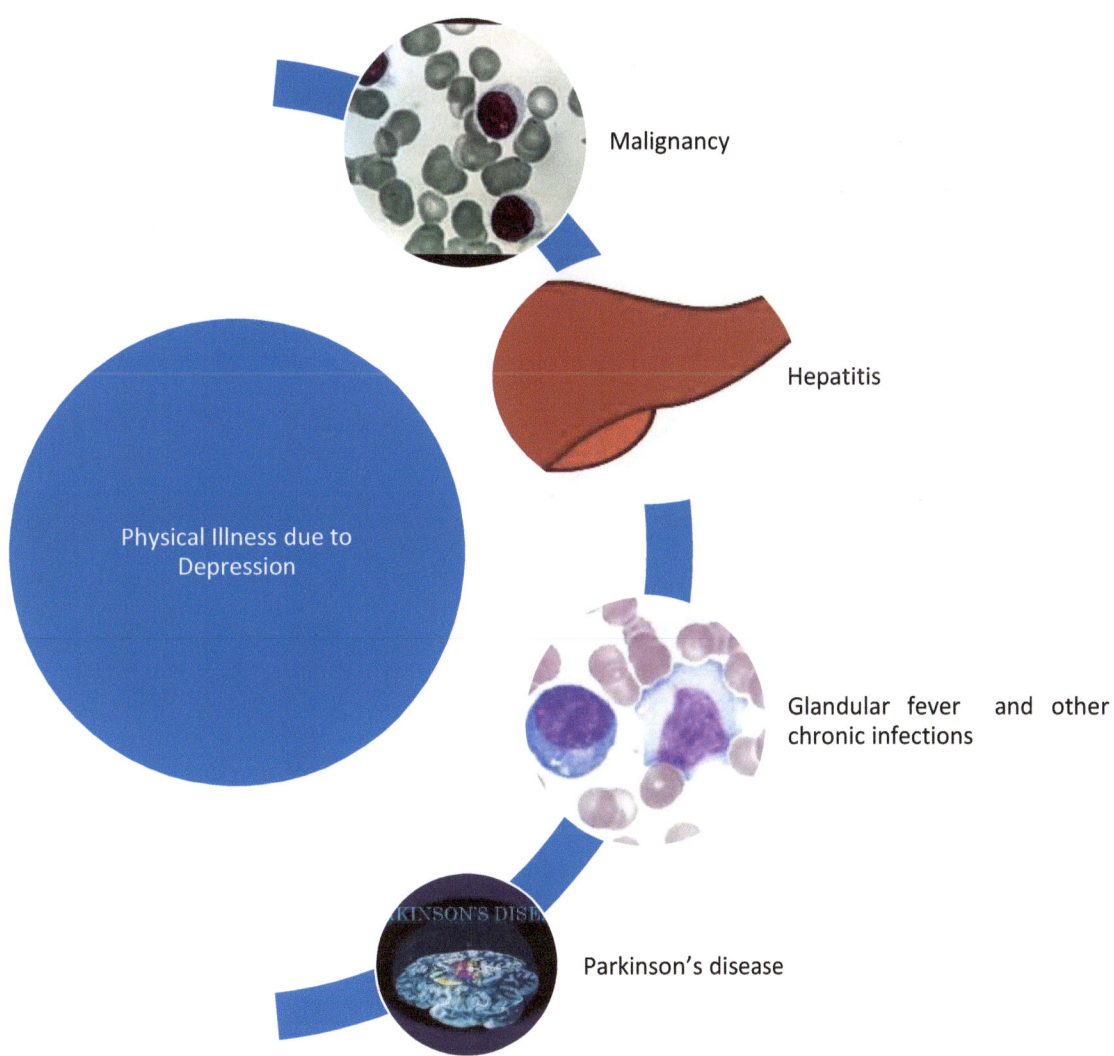

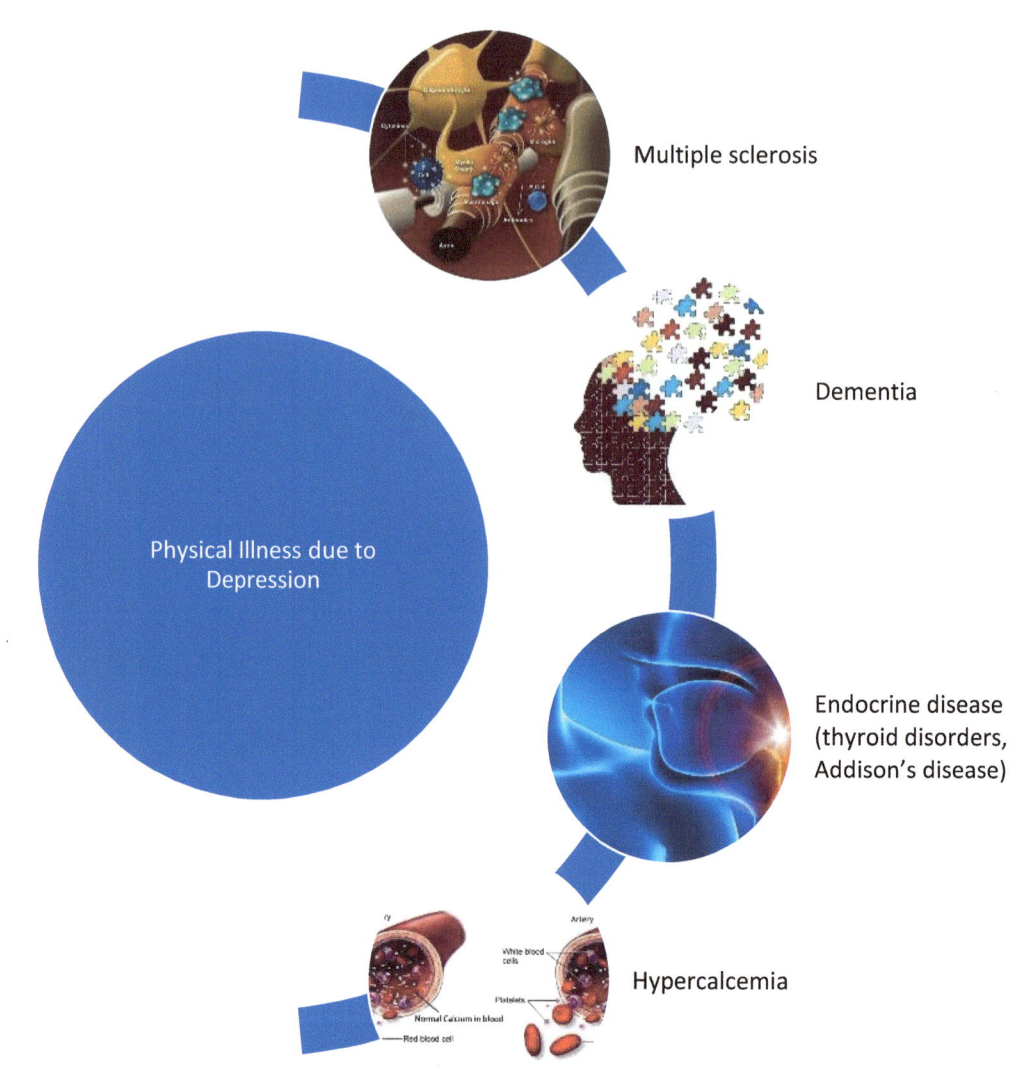

Physical Illness due to Depression

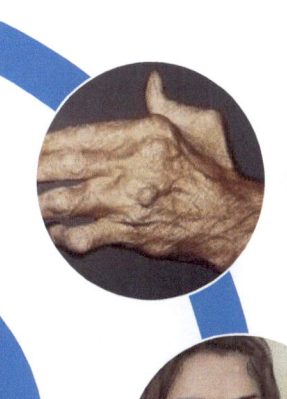
Rheumatoid arthritis

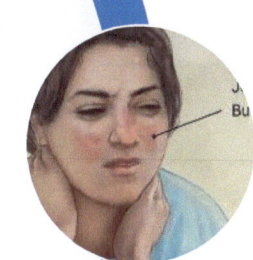
Systemic lupus erythematosus (SLE)

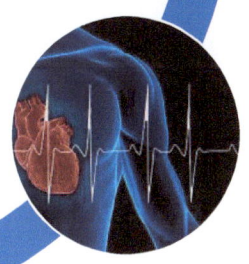
Cardio and cerebrovascular disease

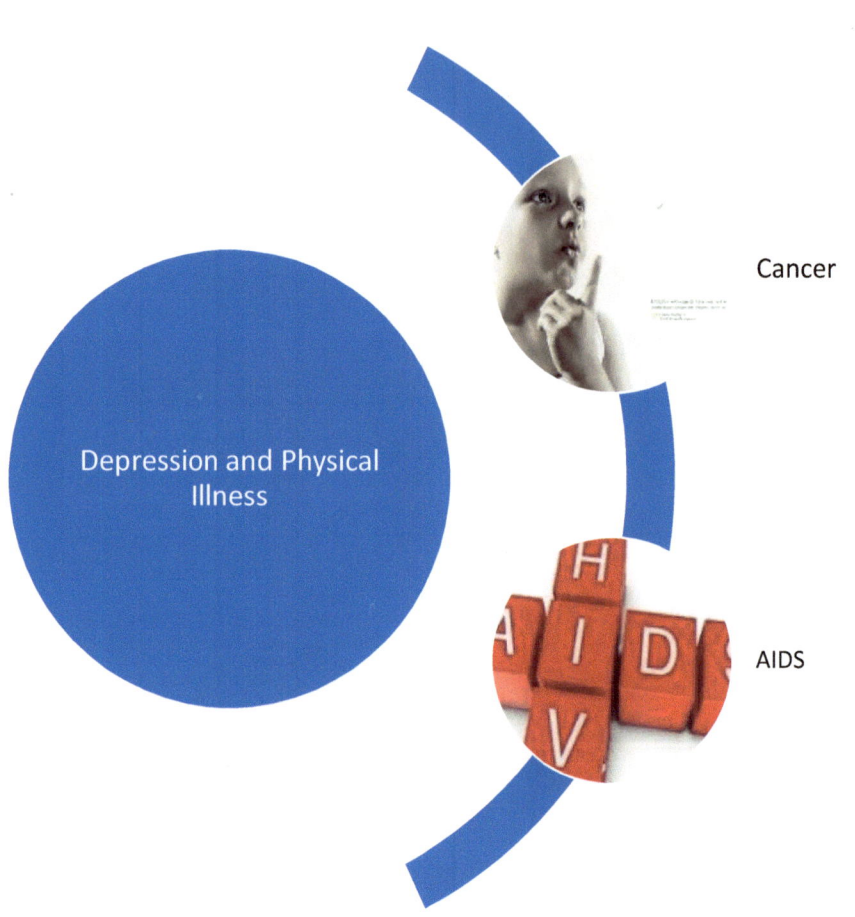

Depression and Physical Illness

Cancer

AIDS

Patients who are taking following medicines can also suffer from Depression:

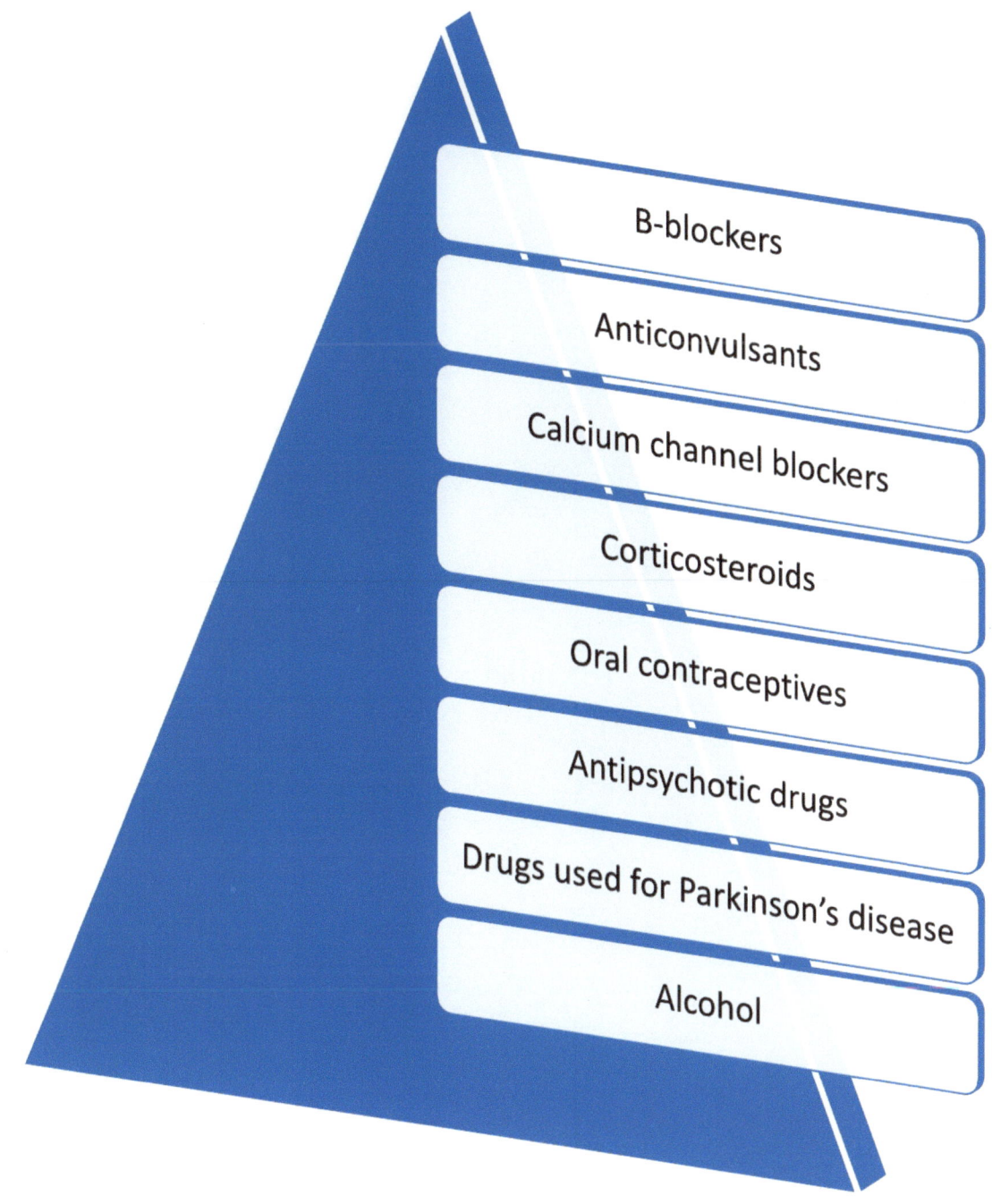

- B-blockers
- Anticonvulsants
- Calcium channel blockers
- Corticosteroids
- Oral contraceptives
- Antipsychotic drugs
- Drugs used for Parkinson's disease
- Alcohol

Possible Reason for Lack of recognision of Depression

- Patients ignore depression in themselves
- Blaming depression on cirmumstances regarding it as understanding
- Overlooking of deression in those who are known to have physical illness
- Misdiagnosis of somatic complaints
- Worry about the side effects of medication
- Fear of Stigma of Mental illness

Pharmacotherapy:

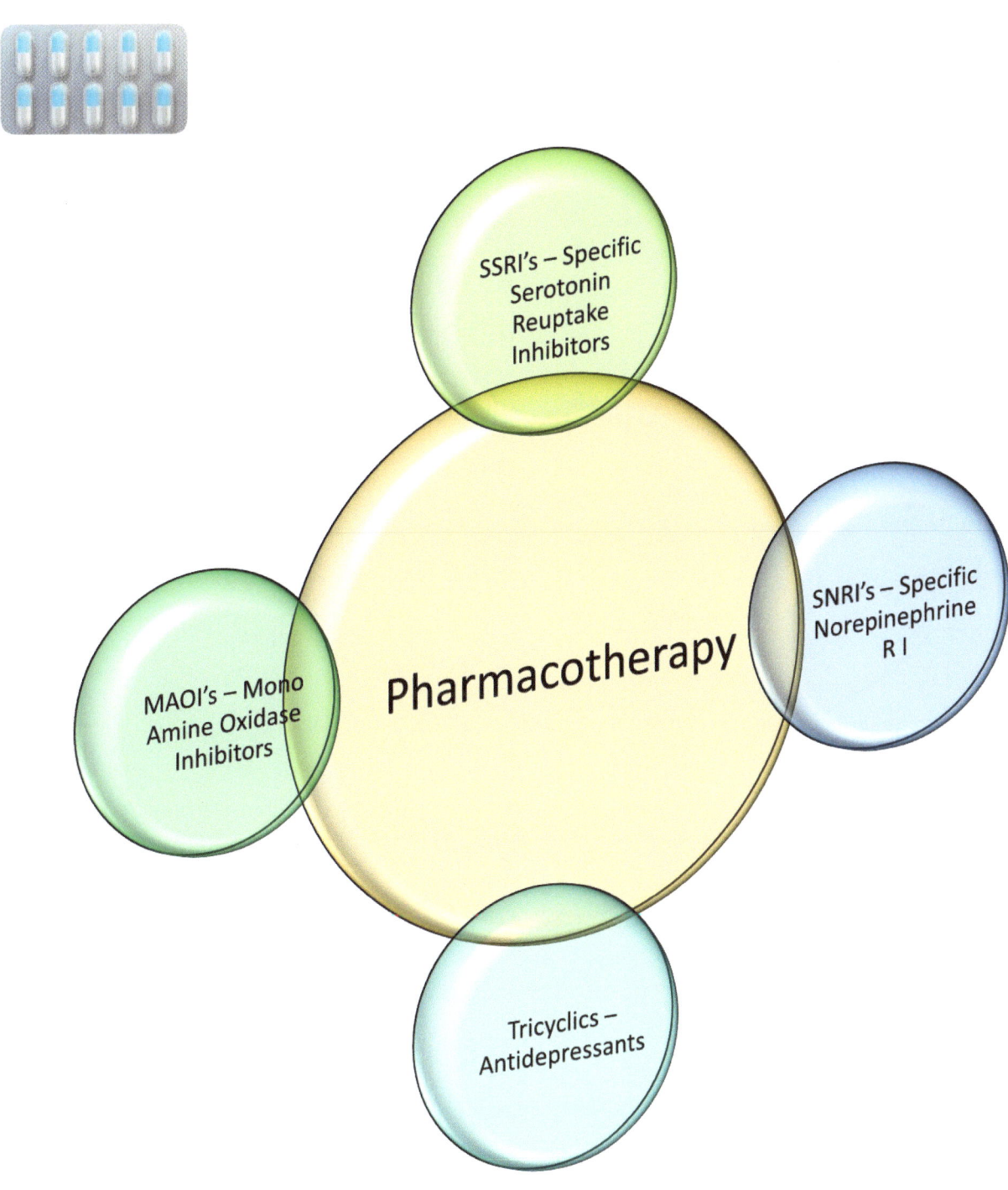

Neurotransmitters And Their Possible Influence On Psychopathology

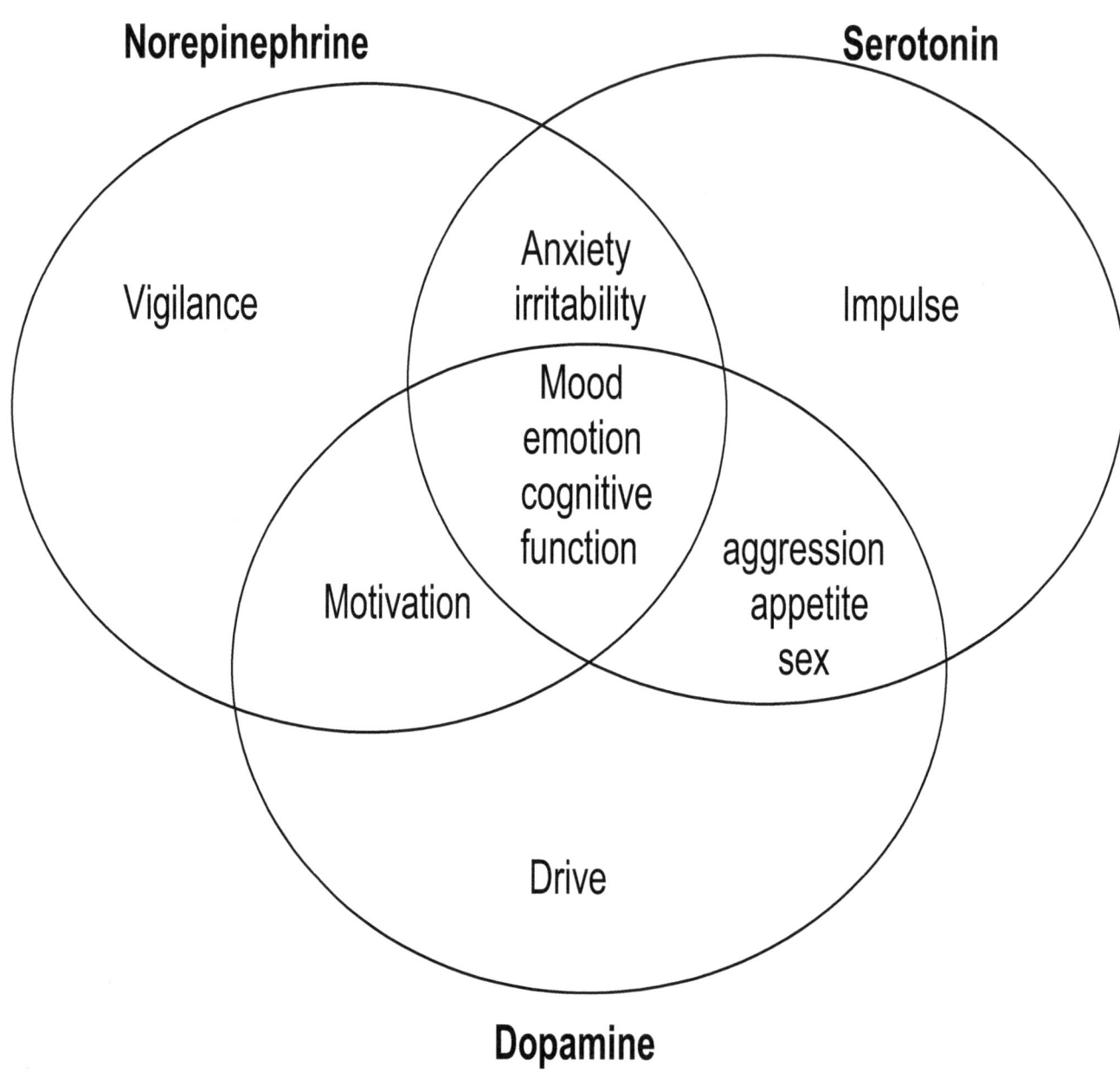

1. **Physical Treatments**

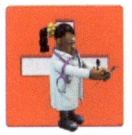

Electroconvulsive (ECT)

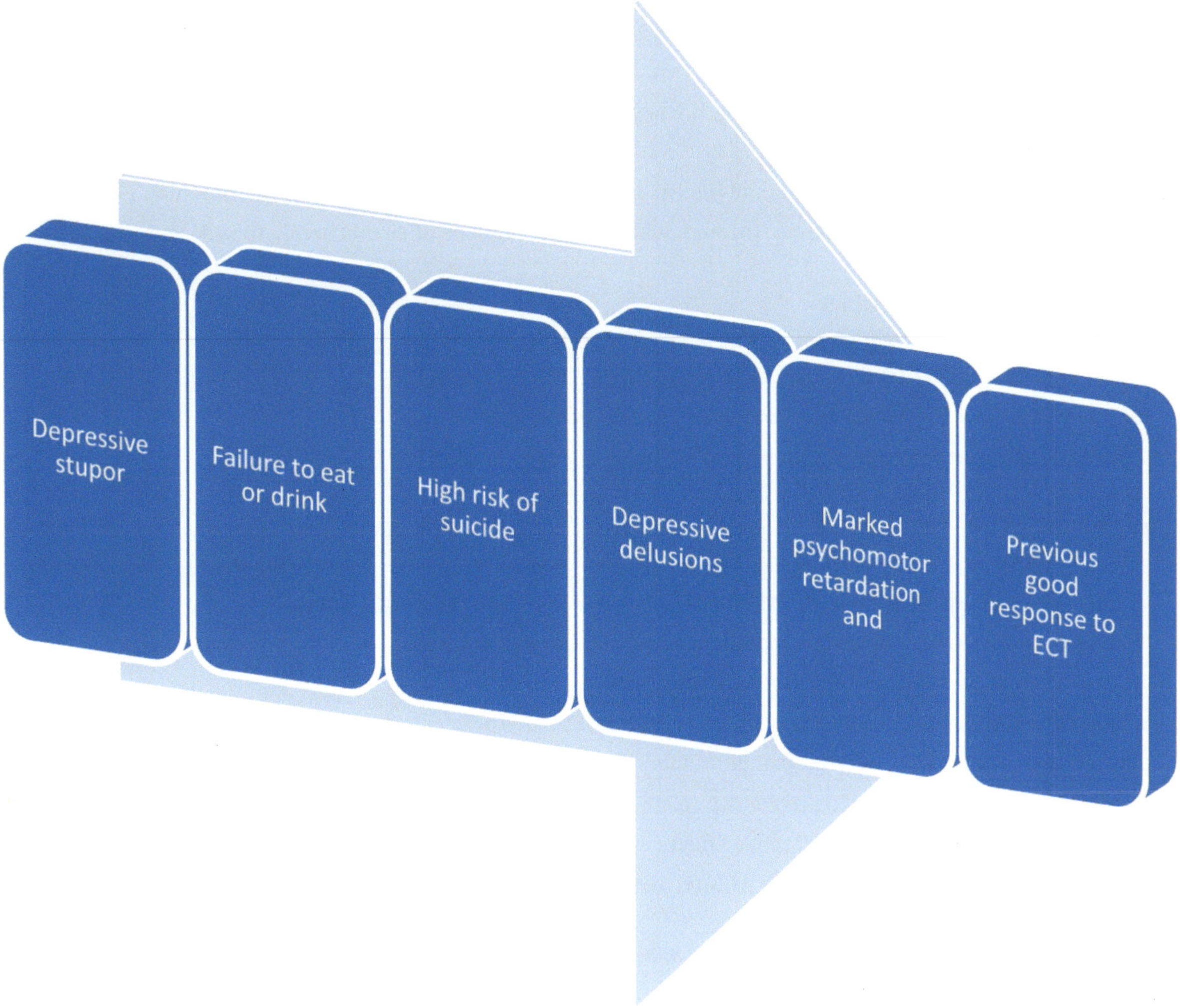

- Depressive stupor
- Failure to eat or drink
- High risk of suicide
- Depressive delusions
- Marked psychomotor retardation and
- Previous good response to ECT

2. **Psychological Treatments:**

Cognitive-Behavior Therapy

Cognitive-behavior therapy (CBT) is one of the most extensively researched and widely adopted psychological treatments for depression. It is based on the assumption that depressive moods are perpetuated and maintained through irrational beliefs and a distorted attitude towards the self, the environment and the future.

Depression is argued to result from cognitions and not mood and postulates that there are three maladaptive elements of depression.

A cognitive triad recurrent negative views that directly shape how the person:
- Sees themselves (negative self-concept, e.g. worthless)
- The world (overestimation of demands, e.g. life is meaningless) and
- The future (e.g. hopeless)
- Irrational schemata based on the past and logical errors that pervade the assessment of oneself and life events; and
- A number of typical processing errors, through which the perceptions of events are distorted

Examples of processing errors include:

- Selective abstraction (attending only to negative aspects of experience);
- Arbitrary inference (jumping to conclusions on inadequate evidence); and
- Over-generalization (making judgments on the basis of single events)

During CBT

- Patients are helped to identify their maladaptive assumptions and processing errors,
- Challenge them by monitoring their experience and associated emotional states
- CBT sessions are standardized and last between 15 and 20 min.
- As 'homework' patients are asked to perform certain tasks, such as keeping a daily record of activities and listing negative thoughts as they occur. This is often complimented by behavioral techniques, such as scheduling pleasurable tasks and breaking seemingly insurmountable problems into smaller, achievable parts.
- Cognitive therapy is particularly effective when combined with antidepressants therapy, and has been found effective in preventing relapse when given in monthly 'booster sessions' after successful acute treatment with antidepressant drugs.

Techniques used in cognitive-behavior therapy for depression:

- Keeping a daily record of activities and negative thoughts
- Monitoring negative thoughts associated with worsening of mood
- Challenging negative thoughts
- Using imagination to 'replay' events
- Questioning the assumptions that lead to negative thoughts
- Planning rewarding activities throughout the day
- Praising oneself for achievements

- Dividing complex tasks into achievable components
- Anticipating performances in challenging situations

Chapter-3: Suicide Risk Assessment

SIMPLESTEPS ASSESSMENT

Suicide is man's way of telling God, 'You can't fire me - I quit!" — Bill Maher

Suicide is the act of killing yourself, most often as a result of depression or other mental illness.

[1]Suicide is ultimate solution of any problem. It does solve your problem. Like if you die, your problems do get ended because problem for you gets finished after once you die.

[2]Emile Durkheim classified different types of suicides based on different types of relationship between the actor and his society.

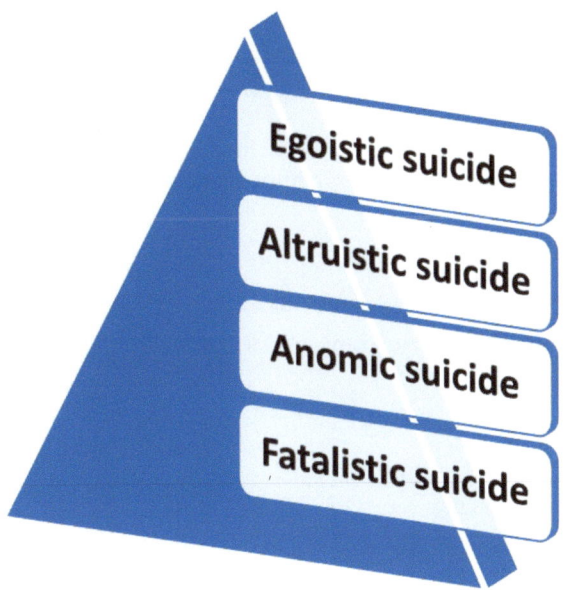

(1) Egoistic suicide:

According to Durkheim, when a man becomes socially isolated or feels that he has no place in the society he destroys himself. This is the suicide of self-centred person who lacks altruistic feelings and is usually cut off from mainstream of the society.

(2) Altruistic suicide:

This type of suicide occurs when individuals and the group are too close and intimate. This kind of suicide results from the over integration of the individual into social proof, for example – Sati customs, Dannies warriors.

(3) Anomic suicide:

This type of suicide is due to certain breakdown of social equilibrium, such as, suicide after bankruptcy or after winning a lottery. In other words, anomic suicide takes place in a situation which has cropped up suddenly.

---

[1] Suicide: The forever decision, New 3rd edition, by Dr. Paul Quinnett, Chapter-1
[2] https://courses.lumenlearning.com/atd-bmcc-sociology/chapter/what-are-the-types-of-suicide-given-by-durkheim/

(4) Fatalistic suicide:

This type of suicide is due to overregulation in society. Under the overregulation of a society, when a servant or slave commits suicide, when a barren woman commits suicide, it is the example of fatalistic suicide.

[3]Suicide Risk Assessment:

How to find out whether the person is mentally unstable and there is a probability that h/she can harm himself.

When such case comes to a psychologist then to find out whether the person is having suicidal thought process or not.

To identify this psychologist will perform suicide risk assessment. The suicide risk assessment is set of open and close ended questions which helps us to know whether the person is having thoughts for

1. **Suicidal:**
    a. Are you thinking for killing yourself?
2. **I – Ideation:** Assessing the thought process and an active intent
    a. When did the thoughts begin?
    b. How frequent are they?
    c. Are they obsessive? (playing continuously on mind)
    d. Can you control them?
    e. On a scale of 1-10 how likely are you to commit suicide? 1- Not very likely to kill yourself and 10- very likely to kill
    f. How high/low has it gone?
    g. What made it go that high/low?
    h. What will make it worse?
    i. What will make it better?

3. **M – Method:** Assessing the means of killing self and plan to use those means
    a. Have you thought about a method of killing yourself?
    b. Have you thought about when you would kill yourself?
    c. Have you thought about where you would do it?
    d. Do you have the mean? / Are the means available?

4. **Pain/Perturbation:** Assessing the degree of emotional pain
    a. On a scale of 1-10 how much emotional pain are you in right now?

---

[3] Course material of Hyderabad Academy of Psychology -Director - Diana Monteiro

      b. What would it bring it to10?
      c. What would it bring it to 1?

5. **Loss:** Assessing the experience of perceived or actual loss (integrality/Pride)
   a. Have you lost anything or anyone in the recent past?
   b. Do you anticipate losing anything in the near future?
   c. How has this loss affected you?
   d. How much time do you spend thinking about this loss?

6. **Earlier Attempts:** Assessing previous attempts
   a. Have you ever attempted suicide before?
   b. What happened in the past attempts?
   c. What happened after the attempt?
   d. What happened so that you did not kill yourself?
   e. Did you want to die at the time?

7. **Substance Use:** Assessing current use and compliance with prescription medication
   a. Do you drink alcohol or use drugs?
   b. When suicidal do you drink or use drugs?
   c. How much do you drink/use?
   d. Do you take your medicines as prescribed?
   e. Why not? (stock piling)

8. **Trouble Shooting:** Assesses current problem-solving ability and level of cognitive constriction (tunnel vision)
   a. Are you willing not to kill yourself?
   b. What have you tried in the past to help you with your issues?
   c. What would you be willing to do?
   d. Have you tried everything you can think of to help?
   e. Have you given up?

9. **Emotions and Diagnosis:** Assessing six key suicidal emotions and relationship to mental illness
   a. Hopelessness: do you feel hopeless?
      - How much hope do you have?
   b. Depression
   c. Impulsivity – How impulsive are you?
   d. Helplessness: do you feel helpless
   e. Worthlessness: do you feel worthless
   f. Loneliness: do you feel lonely?

10. **Parental / Family History:** Assess history and prevalence of suicide and mental illness within family
    a. Has anyone in your family attempted or completed suicide?
    b. Is there a family history of mental illness?

  c. Has anyone been hospitalized for mental health?

11. **Stressors and Life Events:** Assess context of current or past life stressor
    a. What is going on in your life that is causing you to think about suicide?
    b. Which of the problems you are facing is more stressful to you?

By this assessing this psychologist will able to find that whether person is thinking for commenting a suicide or not.

Famous stars who committed suicide due to mental illness:

1. **Case: Robin Williams:** A very famous actor, there was no problem related to money in his life. He had name, success and fame. He had received many awards. Still he committed suicide. He is suffering from Lewy Body Disease.[4]

2. **Case: Marilyn Monroe:** Famous star battled with physical & mental health issues resulting committing suicide by taking overdose of barbiturates. She died at a very young age i.e. 36 years.

3. **Case: Kuljeet Randhawa**: famous tv star who committed suicide because of not able to cope up with life pressure & relationship issues.

MENTAL HEALTH PRESENTATION: VOICE PRESENTATION: by Dr. Amit Phillora

https://www.youtube.com/watch?v=UQEglHzsMQA

My Second book Mental health education part 2 will have topics :

- Substance Abuse ;
- Anxiety disorder Management.

---

[4] Lewy body dementia (LBD, sometimes referred to as Lewy body disorder) is an umbrella term that includes Parkinson's disease dementia (PDD) and dementia with Lewy bodies (DLB), two dementias characterized by abnormal deposits of the protein alpha-synuclein in the brain.

Bibliography

1. Baby blues: https://www.youtube.com/watch?v=6kaCdrvNGZw&feature=youtu.be
2. Diagnostic and Statistical Manual of Mental Disorders, 5th Edition: DSM-5 5th Edition by American Psychiatric Association (Author)
3. Anxiety and Depression-Prime Video at Amazon.com: https://www.amazon.com/dp/B01MSBQVGS
4. MENTAL HEALTH PRESENTATION: VOICE PRESENTATION: by Dr. Amit Phillora
5. https://www.youtube.com/watch?v=UQEglHzsMQA
6. Mental Illness by kitty westin: https://www.youtube.com/watch?v=OsRF8xGgbPA&feature=youtu.be

www.ingramcontent.com/pod-product-compliance
Lightning Source LLC
Chambersburg PA
CBHW041317180526
45172CB00004B/1139